Dedicated to:
All the girls and boys out there who need to have surgery.

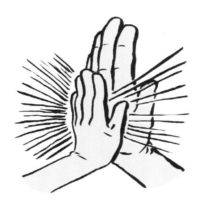

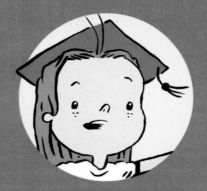

JAKE'S

ACHE

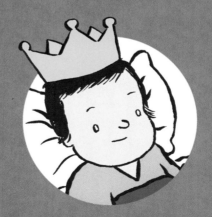

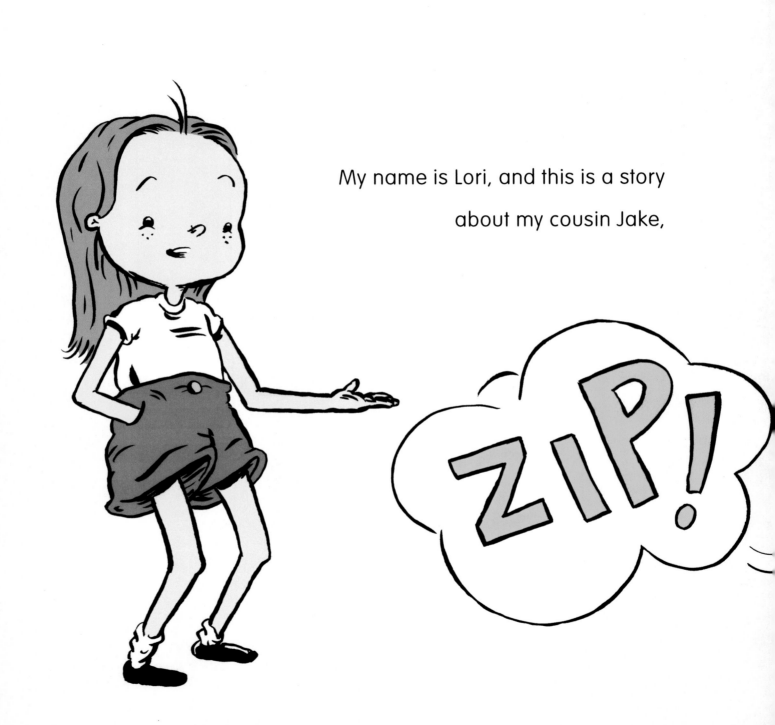

My name is Lori, and this is a story about my cousin Jake,

ZIP!

who was very, very nervous

because he had a

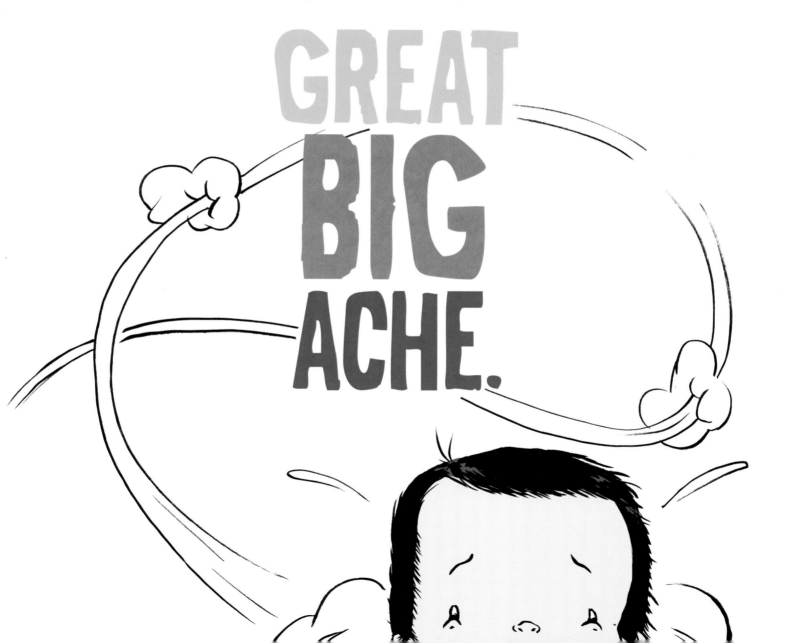

GREAT
BIG
ACHE.

When we found out he needed surgery,

I remembered my own surgery day.

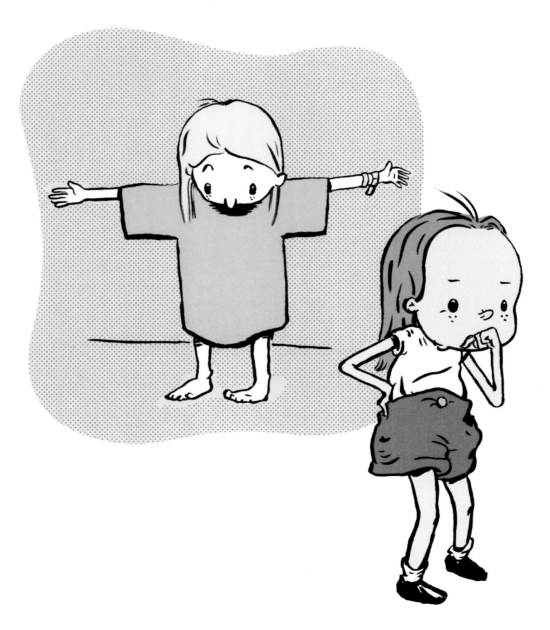

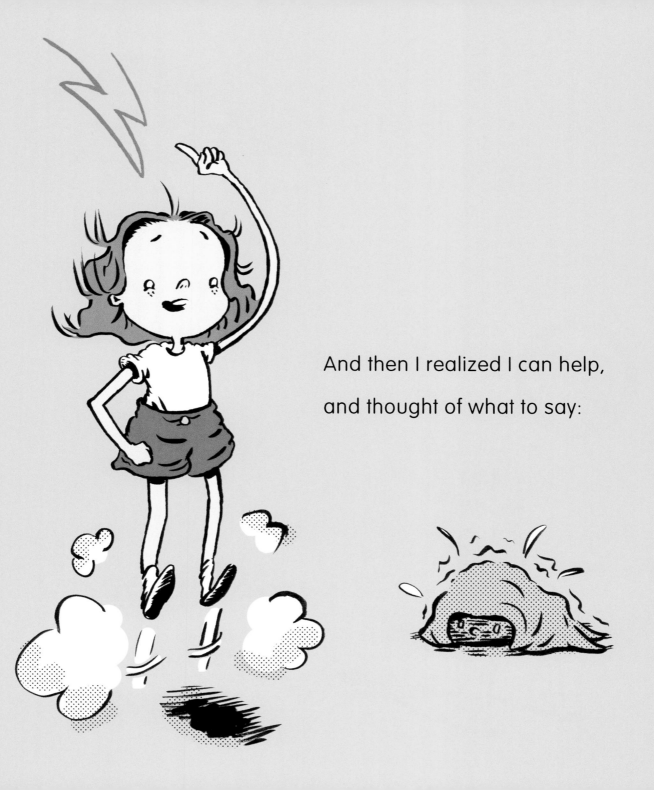

And then I realized I can help,

and thought of what to say:

Don't
be afraid!

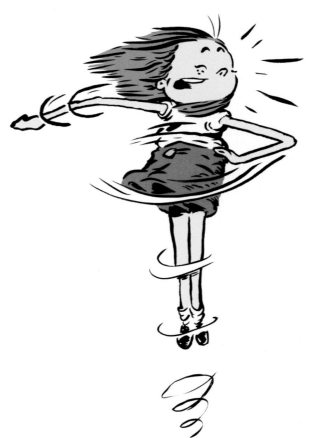

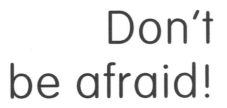

No need to fear!

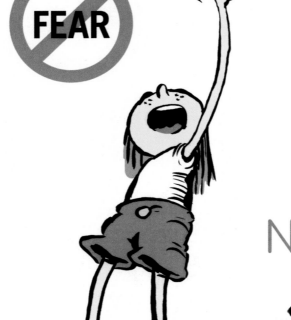

Your oldest, fearless cousin is now right here!

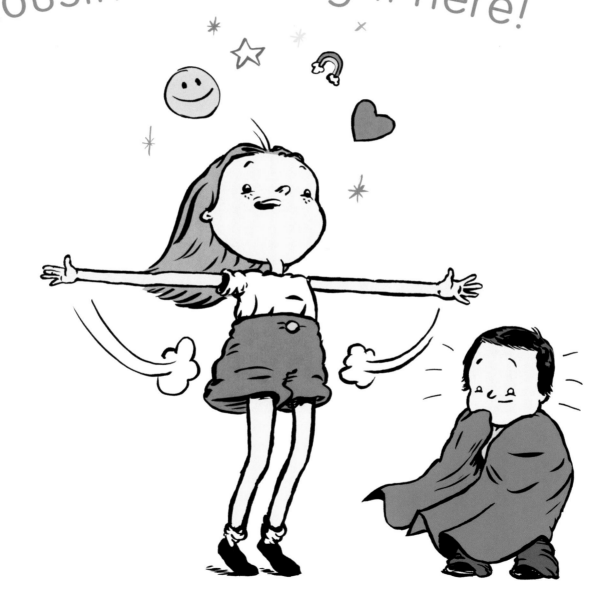

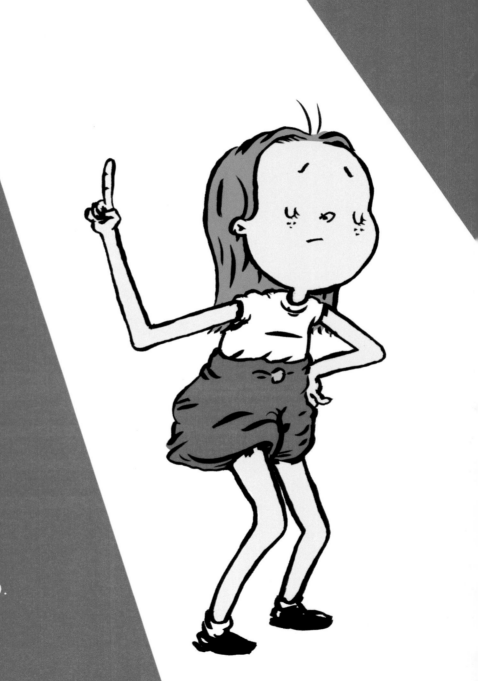

I'm a surgery pro,

and you'll be one too.

If you listen up,

you'll know what to do.

You can't eat before surgery—

that's what they'll say.

You need an empty tummy,

or there will be a long delay.

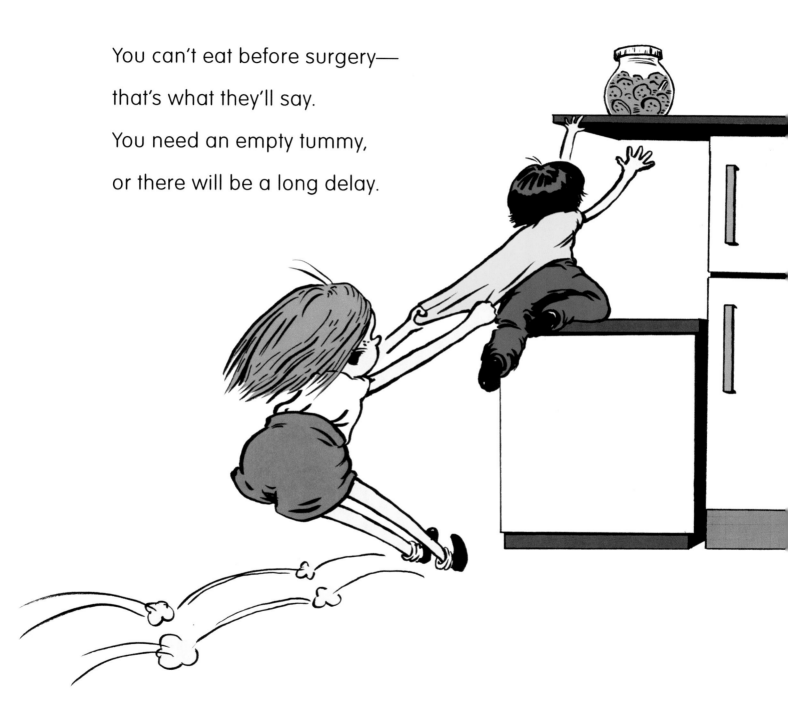

They'll give you a gown,

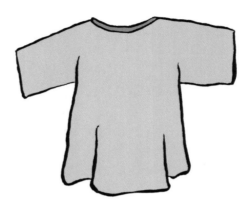

and some soft socks too.

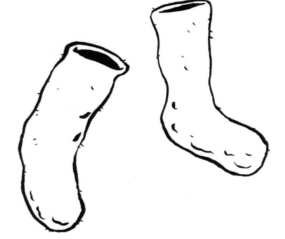

Then it's time to lay down.

(Your blanket may be blue.)

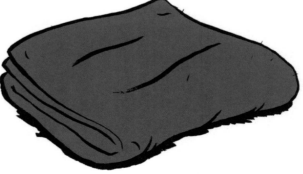

Next, you'll hang out and wait.

You'll stay all cozy and warm.

The nurses, they will check on you.

Don't worry. This is the norm.

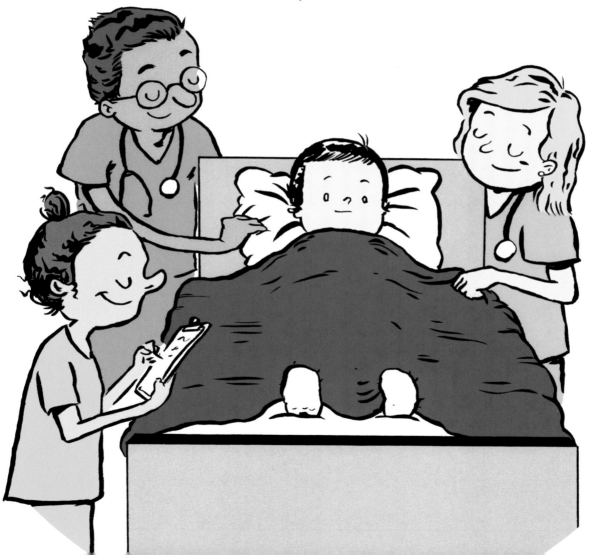

Doctors get dressed for surgery too.

They want everything to be clean.

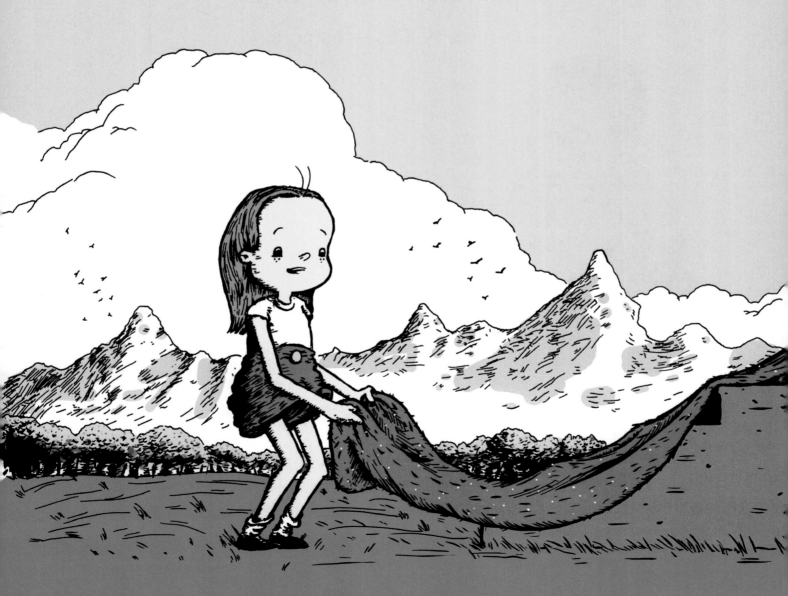

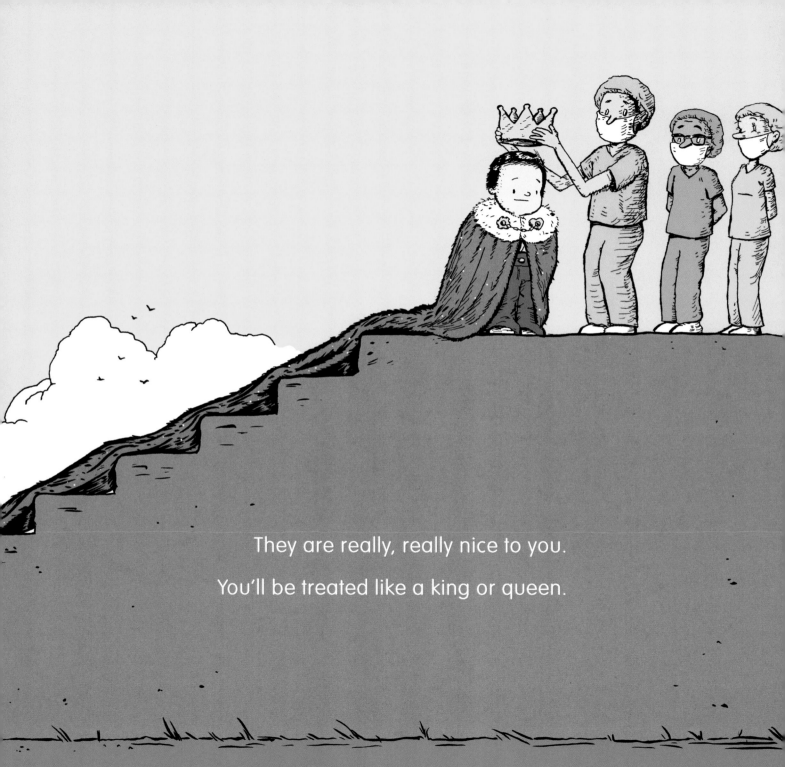

They are really, really nice to you.

You'll be treated like a king or queen.

Mom and Dad will stay nearby.

There is no need to fear.

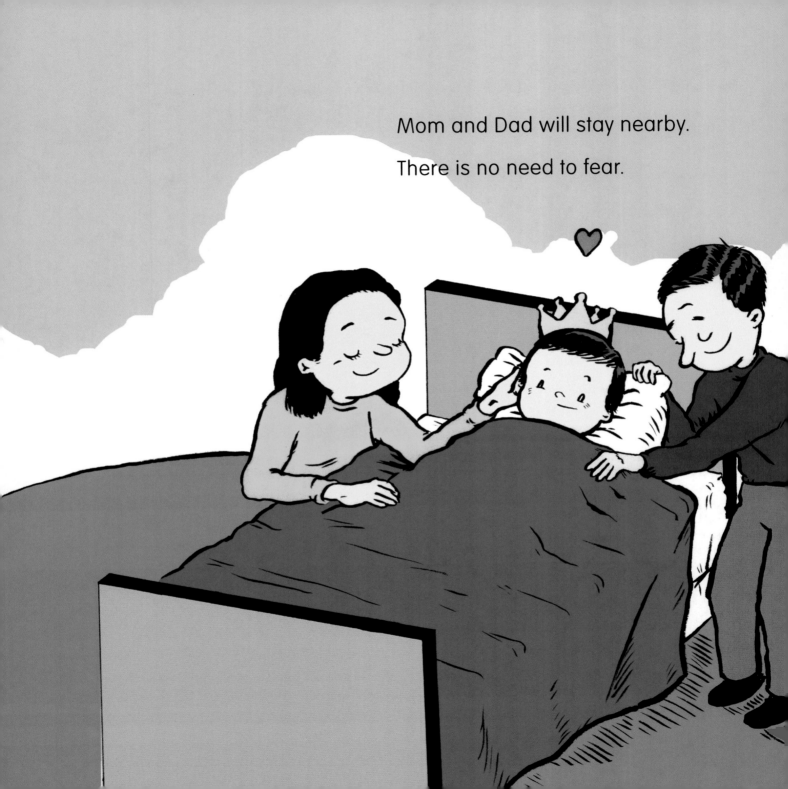

You'll never be alone.

Let me make that perfectly clear.

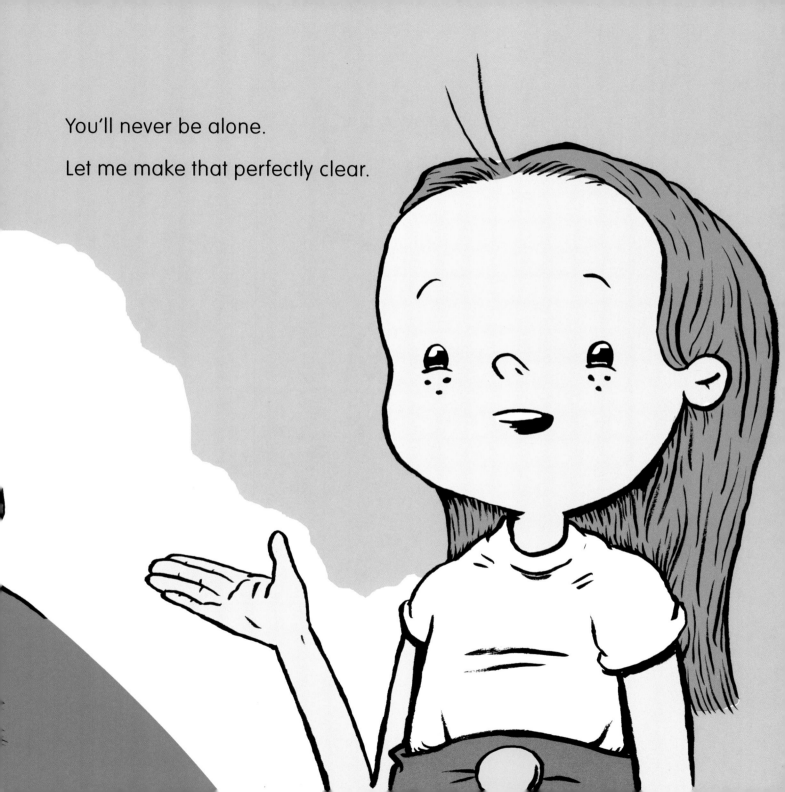

You'll get a thin straw called an IV.

But first you'll feel a pinch.

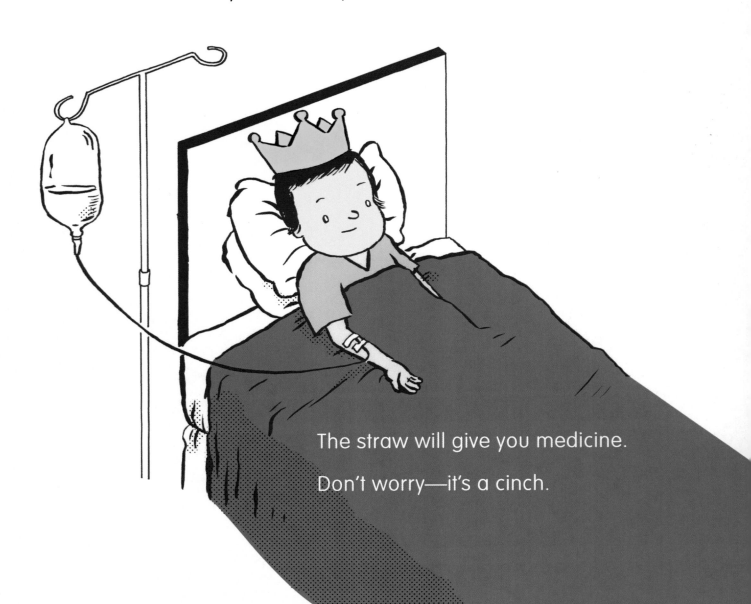

The straw will give you medicine.

Don't worry—it's a cinch.

You'll get wheeled into a room

with loads and loads of light.

That's where you get surgery.

Don't worry—the doctors don't bite.

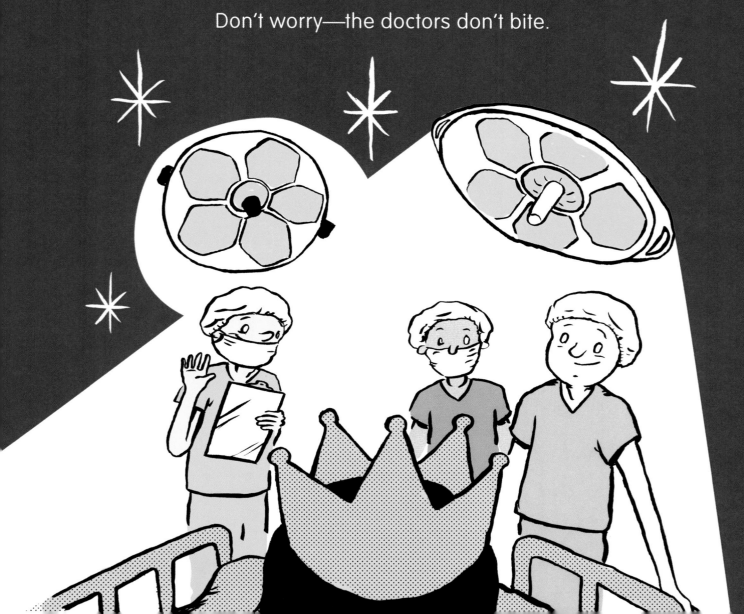

You'll get a little sleepy.

From the medicine, you will rest.

The nurses are extraordinary.

The doctors are the best.

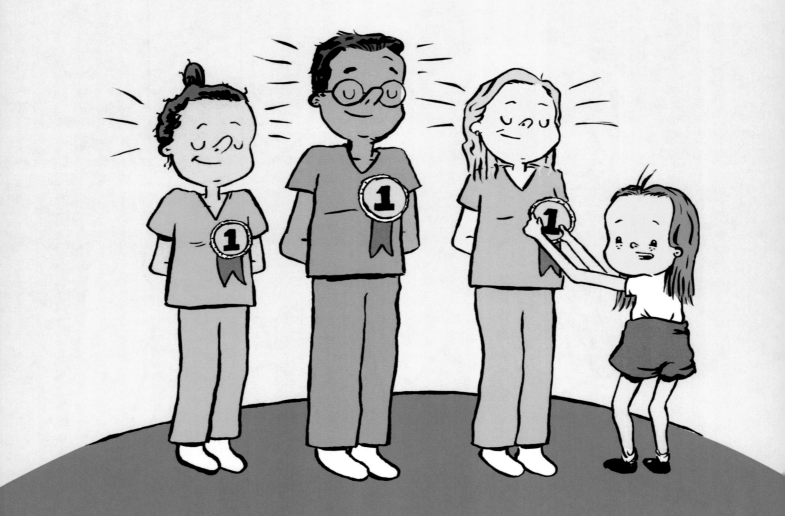

Whether it's tonsils,

an ear, or even a knee.

Let me get to the point—

you'll have to trust me.

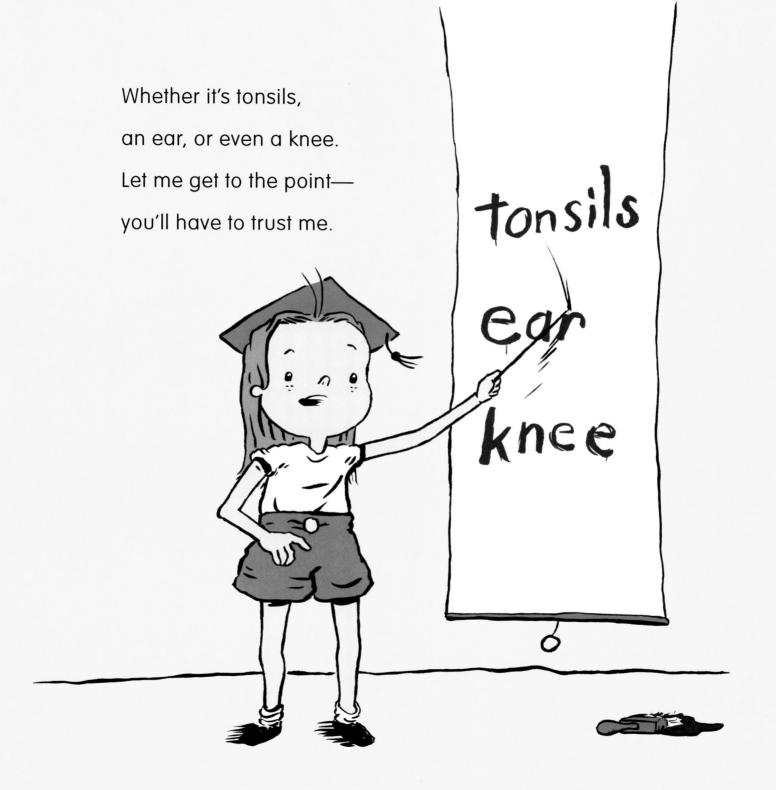

Surgery can seem scary.

It's okay to feel that way.

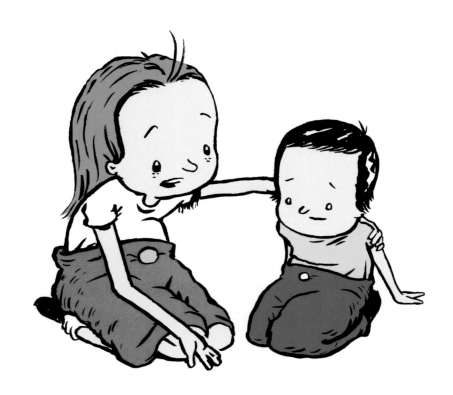

But it goes by very quickly.

And I promise—it'll be okay.

Surgery goes by very fast.

That may be a surprise.

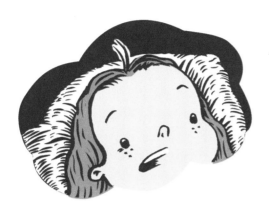

THAT'S ALL?
I'M DONE?

is what I said.

You'll get a big high five!

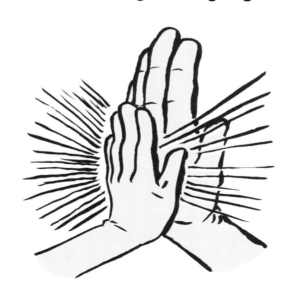

Once your surgery is over,

you will need to rest.

That's what always happens

That's what's always best.

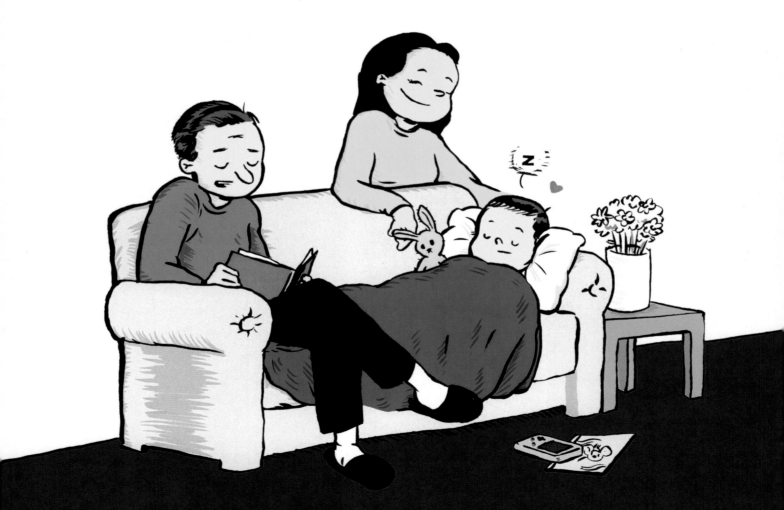

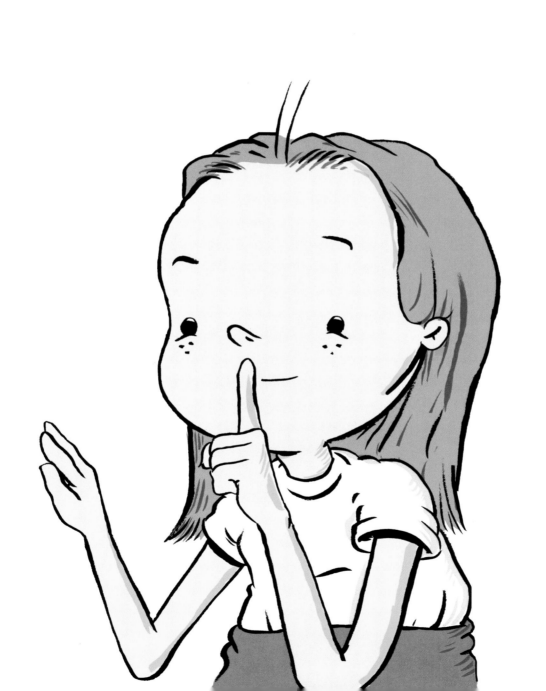

THE END!